Quick Reference Guide to Veterinary Medical Kits

Carole Bowden Dip AVN (Surg) VN
Jo Masters VN

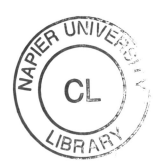
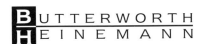

**BUTTERWORTH
HEINEMANN**

An imprint of Elsevier Science

Edinburgh London New York Oxford Philadelphia St Louis Sydney Toronto 2003

BUTTERWORTH-HEINEMANN
An imprint of Elsevier Science Limited
© 2003, Elsevier Science Limited. All rights reserved.

First published 2003

ISBN 0 7506 4959 3

British Library Cataloguing in Publication Data
A catalogue record for this book is available from the
British Library

Library of Congress Cataloging in Publication Data
A catalog record for this book is available from the
Library of Congress

Notice
Medical knowledge is constantly changing. Standard safety precautions
must be followed, but as new research and clinical experience broaden
our knowledge, changes in treatment and drug therapy may become
necessary or appropriate. Readers are advised to check the most current
product information provided by the manufacturer of each drug to be
administered to verify the recommended dose, the method and duration
of administration, and contradictions. It is the responsibility of the
practitioner, relying on experience and knowledge of the patient,
to determine dosages and the best treatment for each individual patient.
Neither the Publisher nor the author assumes any liability for any injury
and/or damage to persons or property arising from this publication.

The Publisher

your source for books,
journals and multimedia
in the health sciences

www.elsevierhealth.com

The
publisher's
policy is to use
**paper manufactured
from sustainable forests**

Printed in China

Contents

Introduction

The aim of this book is to provide an easy reference point for those veterinary staff who are involved with medical nursing procedures. It is not intended to be used as a textbook but as a handy guide that can be kept in the preparation room for easy referral.

This guide will be invaluable to both student veterinary nurses preparing for a specific procedure for the first time and to veterinary staff anticipating an unfamiliar medical nursing procedure.

Each section is designed to cover the basic range of equipment necessary for routine medical procedures; however, flexibility for individual preferences should be assumed.

1
General medical nursing

Records

Efficient nursing of the medical case requires a thorough understanding of the methods of preventing the spread of infection, the ability to recognize the normal from the abnormal and dedication to recording the patient's progress throughout the treatment.

Record keeping is an absolute priority. Records should be constantly updated and referred to regularly. In addition to the owner and patient details, the basic parameters that should be recorded include:

- temperature
- pulse
- respiration
- urination
- defecation
- appetite
- type of food
- fluid intake
- drugs
- demeanour.

Examples of specific record types include:

- observation
- hospitalization
- nursing protocols
- fluid balance
- nutritional support.

To avoid any confusion, records should stay with the patient at all times whilst in the surgery. Ideally, all records should be stored for a minimum of 2 years (recommended by the Veterinary Defence Society).

OBSERVATION RECORD										
PATIENT ID				CLINICAL HISTORY						
SPECIES & BREED										
AGE **SEX** **WEIGHT**										
VETERINARY SURGEON										
VETERINARY NURSE										
MONITOR & RECORD EVERY .... DAILY										
DATE & TIME	T	P	R	MM CRT	DEMEANOUR	FLUID TYPE & DRIP RATE	FLUID INPUT	FLUID/URINE OUTPUT	WEIGHT	MEDICATION	COMMENT

Figure 1.1. Example of an observation sheet.

Kennel Chart

Animal	Owner	Case Number
Species	Clinician	Student
Breed	Clinical Summary	
Colour		
Sex		
Age		

Date	Day No.	Date	Day No.
Weight	Diet	Weight	Diet

	AM	PM		AM	PM
Temp			Temp		
Pulse			Pulse		
Resp			Resp		
Fed			Fed		
Ate			Ate		
Drank			Drank		

Taken Out				Taken Out			
Urine				Urine			
Faeces				Faeces			

MEDICATION		MEDICATION	
PROCEDURES		PROCEDURES	
COMMENTS		COMMENTS	

Figure 1.2. Example of a hospitalization sheet.

DIABETIC PATIENT
Diabetes mellitus

DAILY PROTOCOL

KEEP TO THE SAME FOOD, INSULIN AND EXERCISE REGIME UNLESS
INSTRUCTED OTHERWISE

Morning • Collect urine sample and test with Clinitest kit (at walk or from litter tray)
         • Record result and check insulin dose with V/S
         • Administer Insulin
         • Feed one third of daily food

Afternoon • Eight hours after insulin/first feed, Obtain blood sample
            Test with Dextrostix or Vettest, Record result
          • Feed two thirds of food

COMPLICATIONS
Hypoglycaemia
HAS THE ANIMAL HAD INSULIN? IF SO WHEN?
SIGNS = Drowsiness, weakness, ataxia, collapse
ACTION = Contact V/S
         One/Two tablespoon of honey on tongue
         Prepare equipment for blood sample collection
         Prepare Glucose for I/V administration 5% Dextrose 10–12 ml/kg I/V.
         RECORD ACTIONS

FLUID THERAPY PROTOCOL

PREPARE ALL EQUIPMENT IN ADVANCE AND WEIGH THE ANIMAL
CHOOSE YOUR FLUIDS!!

Daily fluid requirements = 50 ml/kg/24 h
                          = 25 ml Urinary loss + 25 ml Faecal/Respiratory loss
Vomit loss   = 2 ml/kg/vomit
Diarrhoea loss   = 4 ml/kg/explosion!

Example • 10 kg dog anorexic
          10 kg × 50 ml per 24 h = 500 ml   500 ml over 8 h
                                  = 20 ml/h   = 62.5 ml/h
                                  = 0.3 ml/min   = 1.04/min

          Average giving set delivers 20 drops per ml (delivery over 8 h)
                    5 kg requiring 250 ml = 1 drop/5 s
                   10 kg requiring 500 ml = 1 drop/3 s
                   20 kg requiring 1000 ml = 1 drop/1.5 s
                   30 kg requiring 1500 ml = 1 drop/0.75 s
          Where possible monitor urine volume passed – minimum 1 ml/kg/h

CATHETER CARE • Ensure catheter is placed aseptically and maintained
                 aseptically
               • Keep catheter covered to prevent patient interference/
                 buster collar
               • Flush catheter via giving set port four times daily
                 (minimum) use drip fluid or heparinized saline
               • If unable to unblock catheter prepare equipment
                 ready for new catheter placement
                 RECORD ALL FLUID ADMINISTRATION AND ACTIONS

Figure 1.3. Example of nursing protocols.

NAME: ————————————

CASE NUMBER: ————————————

DATE & TIME	FLUID OFFERED	FLUID INTAKE	I/V FLUID	DRIP RATE

Figure 1.4. Example of a fluid balance record.

SMALL ANIMAL NUTRITION SHEET

CLIENT NAME	ADMISSION DATE	VETERINARY SURGEON
PATIENT NAME	AGE	
SEX	WEIGHT	VETERINARY NURSE

CONDITION

Emaciated	☐	....
Underweight	☐	....
Correct for breed	☐	**MEDICAL/SURGICAL PROBLEMS**
Overweight	☐	1. 3.
Grossly obese	☐	2. 4.

RESTING ENERGY REQUIREMENT (RER)

    RER kcal/day   **Dogs** over 5 kg = $(30 \times kg) + 70$

                  Dogs and cats 5 kg and under = $(60 \times kg) + 70$

ILLNESS ENERGY REQUIREMENT (IER)

Cage rest/hospitalization	1.2	× RER	☐	**RER =** kcal/day
Post surgery	1.2	× RER	☐	
Cachexia/trauma	1.3	× RER	☐	
Sepsis/cancer	1.5	× RER	☐	
Head trauma/major burn	1.7	× RER	☐	**IER =** kcal/day

    IER = RER × ....

DIETARY RECOMMENDATIONS

Protein	☐	Fat	☐
Fibre	☐	Other	☐

    SELECTED FOOD ....

    CALORIFIC DENSITY ....

    AMOUNT TO FEED DAILY = $\dfrac{IER}{Calorific\ density}$ **OR**

Amount =	ml/day
Amount =	g/day

FOOD DOSAGE + ROUTE

DAY 1

DAY 2

DAY 3

PLAN

Continue diet for:	2 weeks	Post surgery
	2–4 weeks	Trauma
	4–12 weeks	Head trauma/burns
	months	Chronic disease/neoplasia

Continue .... diet   for .... weeks.

Figure 1.5. Example of a nutritional support record.

2
General medical nursing

Prevention of the spread of disease – terminology

- **Carrier** – an animal that carries a disease without showing any clinical signs
- **Contagious** – a disease that can be transmitted from one animal to another either by direct or indirect contact
- **Direct contact** – disease is spread as a result of animals coming into physical contact with one another, e.g. biting
- **Fomite** – an inanimate object that can spread disease, e.g. litter tray, bowl
- **Host** – passes disease from itself to a susceptible animal
- **Incubation** – the period between the animal coming into contact with a pathogen and the appearance of clinical disease
- **Indirect contact** – disease is passed without animals coming into physical contact, e.g. via fomites
- **Isolation** – separation of potential vectors from susceptible animals
- **Pathogen** – a disease-causing microorganism, e.g. bacteria
- **Vector** – animate carriers of disease

3
General medical nursing

Hygiene requirements

The prevention of the spread of disease will rely on good basic hygiene protocols. These will apply to the:

- environment
- patient
- personnel.

Basic hygiene protocols

The environment
- All kennels/cages should be cleaned and disinfected on a daily basis.
- All surfaces and equipment should be cleaned and disinfected on a daily basis.
- Bedding must be washed and disinfected between patients.
- All waste must be disposed of correctly.
- All kennel areas should be treated for parasites routinely.

NB. *All surfaces must be cleaned thoroughly before they can be disinfected. The disinfectant of choice must be appropriate for the situation and made up freshly to the correct dilution.*

The patient
- All patients should be housed separately.
- Ideally, all patients should be vaccinated and treated for parasites before being admitted.

- The patient should stay in the same kennel throughout its stay and utilize the same equipment, i.e. bowls, litter trays.
- All patient waste should be promptly removed and disposed of.
- The patient should be kept clean and free of discharges.

Personnel
The prevention of the spread of zoonotic disease is the responsibility of all practice personnel. Common zoonotic diseases include:

- dermatophytosis
- *Echinococcus granulosus*
- leptospirosis
- rabies
- salmonellosis
- sarcoptic mange
- *Toxocara canis*
- toxoplasmosis.

Practice personnel can also act as vectors of disease from animal to animal; therefore, to protect both humans and animals a strict hygiene policy should be implemented. This should include:

- a high standard of personal hygiene, i.e. clean hair (either short or tied back), short nails, no jewellery and clean uniform
- wearing protective clothing at all times, e.g. disposable gloves and apron
- washing hands after touching any animal, even if gloves have been worn
- discarding disposable clothing after use
- not allowing animals to lick the face or mouth
- keeping all animal food preparation equipment separate from human utensils and crockery, and using a separate area for washing these items
- keeping personal vaccinations up to date and seeking medical advice if there is a concern about possible exposure to zoonotic disease.

Isolation and barrier nursing
When patients are placed in isolation, high standards of barrier nursing are essential.

- Ideally, staff members allocated to work on isolation should not be involved with the nursing of any other patients.
- A foot bath containing a suitable disinfectant should be available at the entrance to the isolation facility. This should be freshly prepared at regular intervals.
- Protective clothing should be available at the entrance to the isolation unit. In addition to the usual personal hygiene protocol, foot covers/boots, surgical masks and facilities for their disposal on exit should be made available.
- Each kennel/cage should have its own labelled equipment such as bowls, bedding etc., and these should all be washed and disinfected separately to equipment from other patients.
- Kennels should be cleaned starting with the patient that has the lowest risk of contagion finishing with the patient that is the most likely to spread infection.

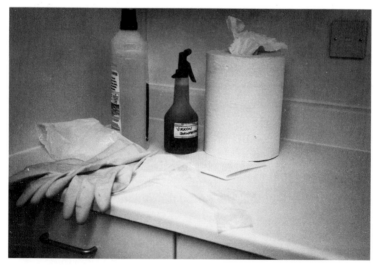

Figure 3.1. Kennel cleaning equipment.

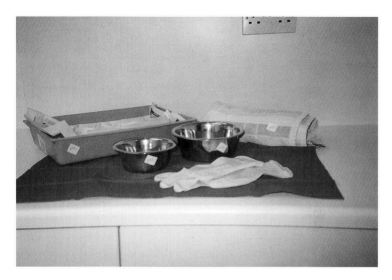

Figure 3.2. Isolation kennels – labelled equipment.

- All cleaning equipment and bedding should be disposable.
- On exiting the isolation facility all protective clothing should be disposed of and hands thoroughly washed.

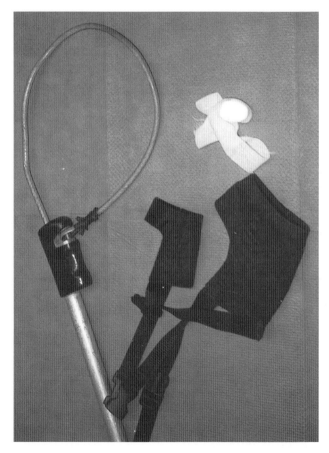

Figure 4.1. Restraint aids (dog catcher, muzzles, white open weave bandage).

4
Medical nursing kits

Examination kits

Restraint aids

One or a combination of the following may be used.

Dogs
- quiet environment
- suitable assistance for size of dog
- personal protective clothing as required
- slip lead
- muzzle
- dog catcher.

Cats
- quiet environment
- suitable assistance, either one or two assistants
- personal protective clothing as required, e.g. gloves, long sleeves
- towel
- crush cage
- cat catcher.

NB. *Drugs can only be used as restraint aids when prescribed by a veterinary surgeon.*

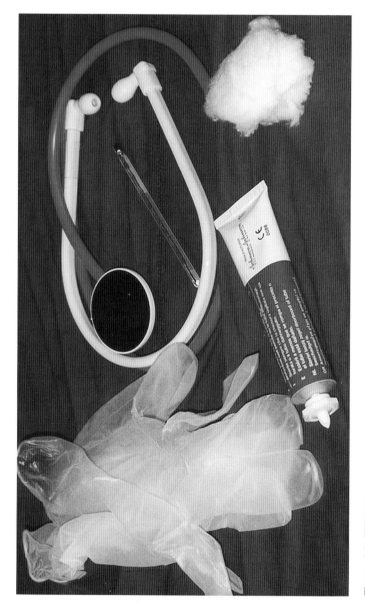

Figure 4.2. TPR kit (gloves, stethoscope, thermometer, cotton wool, lubricant).

Temperature, pulse and respiration

- watch with second hand
- disposable gloves and apron
- an assistant may be required to restrain the patient
- clean disinfected thermometer – either mercury or digital
- lubricant
- tissue
- availability of clinical waste disposal
- stethoscope – may be used to record heart rate
- pen and patient record.

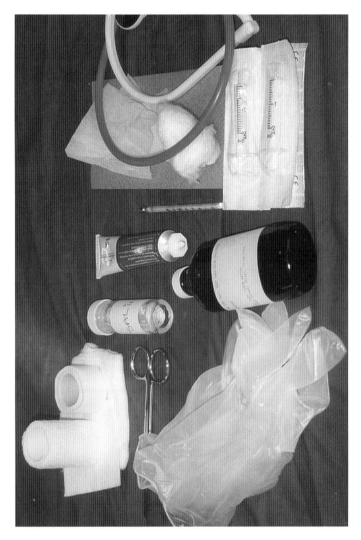

Figure 4.3. In-patient care (gloves, antiseptic, dressings, scissors, thermometer, stethoscope, syringes).

In-patient care

The minimum equipment which should ideally be available in the ward for basic in-patient care could include:

- disposable gloves and aprons
- disposable towel, tissue and cotton wool
- diluted disinfectant solution
- diluted antiseptic solution
- normal saline for bathing external orifices
- a useful range of syringes and needles
- a small range of dressing materials
- scissors
- clean, disinfected thermometers
- lubricant
- stethoscope
- recording facilities, i.e. pens, record sheets
- clean, disinfected basic grooming equipment
- electric clippers
- nail clippers
- clinical waste bin
- sharps container.

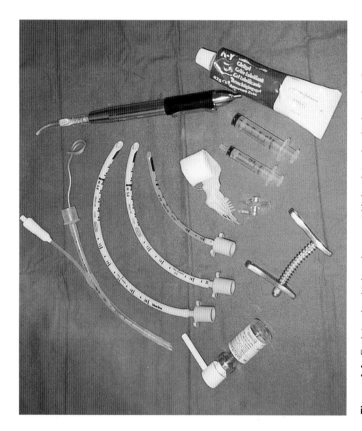

Figure 4.4. Endotracheal tube placement kit (endotracheal tube selection, lubricant, cuff inflator, laryngoscope, tape, mouth gag, local anaesthetic spray).

First aid kits

Airway

Establishing patent airway
1. Endotracheal intubation
    - disposable apron and gloves
    - assistant to restrain patient
    - laryngoscope
    - endotracheal tube
    - lubrication for endotracheal tube
    - white, open weave bandage to tie tube in place
    - cuff inflator
    - mouth gag.

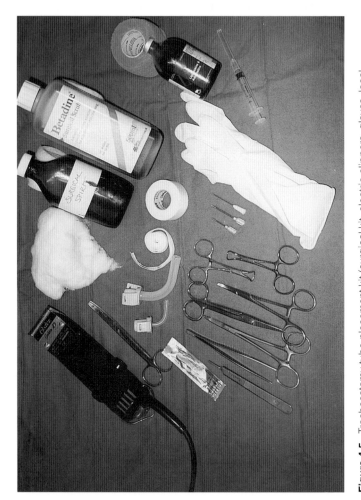

Figure 4.5. Tracheostomy tube placement kit (surgical kit, electric clippers, gloves, local anaesthetic, skin prep. solutions, tracheostomy tubes).

2. Emergency tracheostomy kit
    - assistant to restrain patient
    - electric clippers
    - local anaesthetic
    - surgical skin preparation solution (chlorhexidine or povidine iodine)
    - surgical spirit
    - cotton wool/gauze swabs
    - minor surgical kit – scalpel handle and blade, rat tooth forceps, Mayo scissors and towel clips
    - drape (desirable)
    - tracheostomy tube and tape
    - selection of small uncuffed endotracheal tubes
    - selection of hypodermic needles: 14 g, 16 g and 18 g
    - sterile gloves.

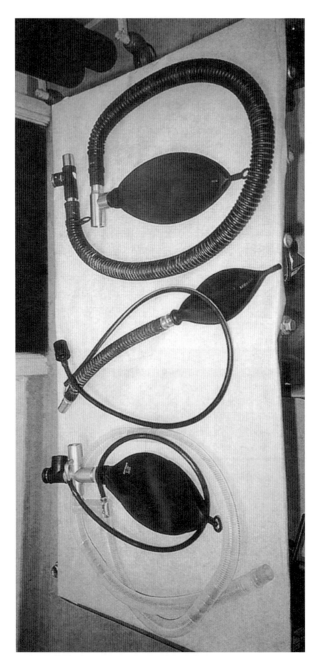

Figure 4.6. IPPV equipment (anaesthetic circuits for IPPV, Bain, Magill Jackson Rees T piece).

Breathing

Supply of oxygen kit
Once a patent airway has been established, provide supply of oxygen using:

- oxygen cylinder and reducing valve
- connector for endotracheal tube
- resuscitation bag
- anaesthetic circuit for intermittent positive pressure ventilation (IPPV) – Ayres T piece with Jackson Rees modification, Bain circuit
- ventilator if available
- oxygen cage/incubator.

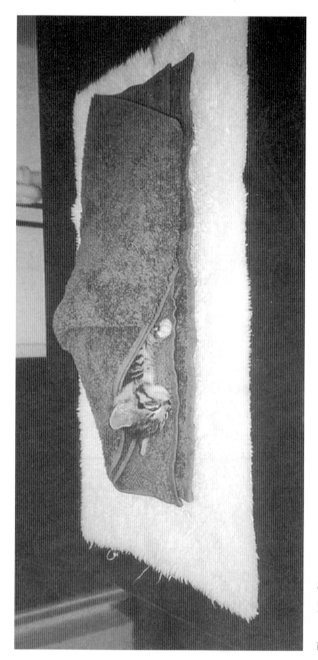

Figure 4.7. Circulatory support kit.

Circulatory support kit

- warm ambient temperature
- heated pads
- hot water bottles wrapped in towels
- blankets
- circulatory support, i.e. fluids
- warmed isotonic fluids
- selection of sterile syringes and needles
- intravenous catheter
- zinc oxide tape
- infusion set
- bung or three-way tap.

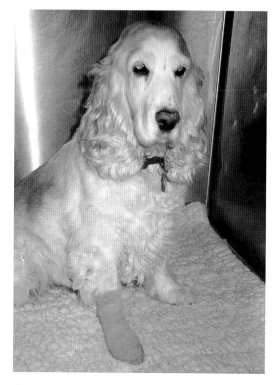

Figure 4.8. Animal recovering from shock.

Shock support kit

- calm, quiet environment
- blankets/bubble wrap/foil wrap
- intravenous fluid solution
- intravenous catheter
- fluid infusion set
- zinc oxide tape
- bung or three-way tap
- record card
- thermometer
- stethoscope
- oxygen supply and masks
- drug therapy as per veterinary surgeon instruction.

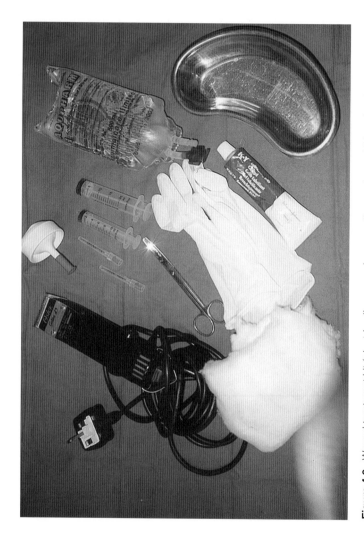

Figure 4.9. Wound treatment kit (electric clippers, scissors, saline, syringes, kidney bowl, gloves, cotton wool, lubricant, wound gel).

Wound treatment kit

- disposable apron and gloves
- kidney bowl
- selection of sterile needles and syringes
- electric clippers
- curved or flat scissors
- wound gels
- sterile dressing/gel
- conforming bandage
- padding/absorbent layer
- tertiary/protective layer
- Elizabethan collar.

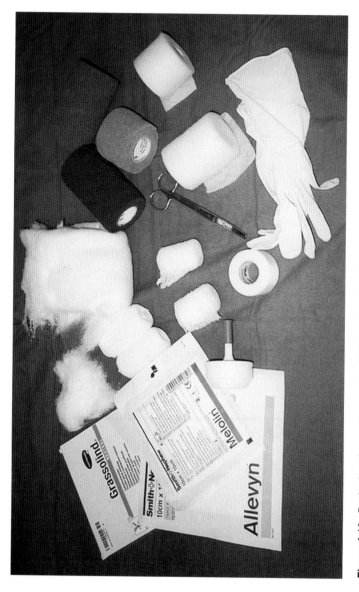

Figure 4.10. Basic dressing and bandaging kit (dressings, bandages, gloves, scissors, swabs, cotton wool).

Bandage and splinting kits

Basic dressing and bandaging kit

- disposable apron and gloves
- curved or flat scissors
- selection of non-adherent dressings
- selection of wound gels
- padding layer – cotton wool, swabs or synthetic padding
- selection of conforming bandage – 5 cm, 7.5 cm and 10 cm
- outer/protective layer bandage – elastic adhesive or self-adhesive conforming bandage – 5 cm, 7.5 cm and 10 cm
- zinc oxide tape.

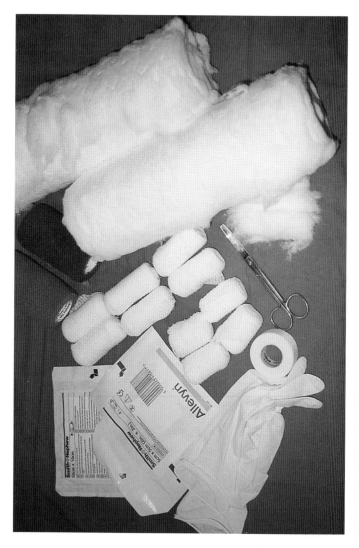

Figure 4.11. RJ bandage kit (dressings, bandages, cotton wool, gloves, scissors).

Robert Jones bandage

- disposable apron and gloves
- curved or flat scissors
- zinc oxide tape
- conforming bandages
- 1–2 cotton wool rolls
- cotton wool to pad between toes
- sterile wound dressing if wound present
- outer protective layer (elastic adhesive or self-adhesive).

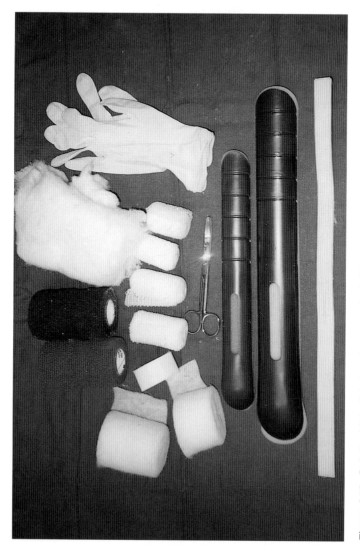

Figure 4.12. Splinting kit (splints, bandages, synthetic foam padding, cotton wool, scissors, gloves).

Splinting kit

- disposable apron and gloves
- scissors/shears to shape/cut splints to size
- selection of splints – gutter, aluminium and foam/polymer gauze
- padding layer – synthetic padding rolls or cotton wool
- sterile dressing if wound present
- cotton wool to pad toes
- selection of conforming bandage
- selection of protective layer bandage – elastic adhesive or self-adhesive.

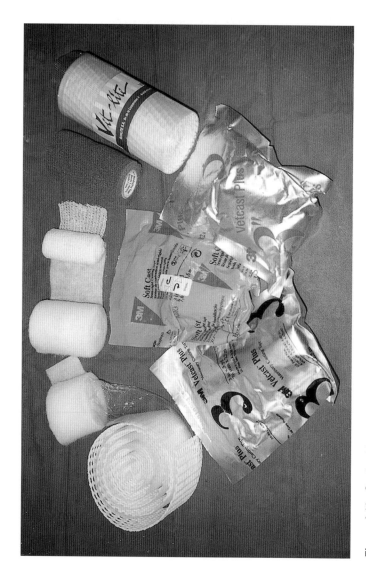

Figure 4.13. Casting kit.

Casting kit

- disposable apron and gloves
- proprietary casting material and instructions
- bowl of water
- paper towel
- padding layer – synthetic or cotton wool
- selection of splints (optional)
- plaster shears or embryotomy wire, handles and rubber tube.

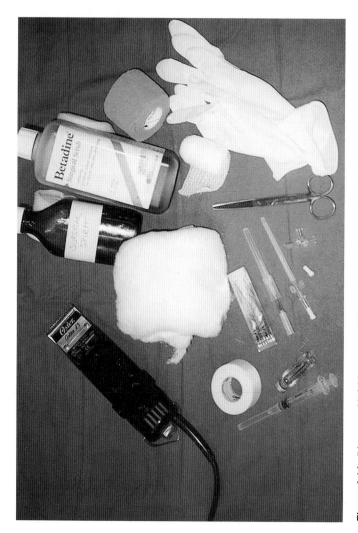

Figure 4.14. IV access kit (skin prep. solutions, gloves, scissors, electric clippers, intravenous catheters, heparinized saline, cotton wool).

Fluid therapy kits

Intravenous access catheter placement kit

This particular kit is suitable for any venepuncture site – cephalic, saphenous or jugular.

- disposable apron and gloves
- electric clippers
- surgical scrub solution – chlorhexidine or povidine iodine
- surgical spirit
- scalpel blade size 11 (optional)
- zinc oxide tapes
- cotton wool swabs
- bung or three-way tap
- heparinized saline
- sterile 21g × 5/8 needle and 2 ml syringe
- intravenous catheter – suitable for patient size (neonate 22–24 g, adult cat and small dog 22–20 g, medium dog 20 g, large dog 18 g)
- needle holders, treves rat tooth forceps, suture needle and suture material to secure catheter (optional/jugular venepuncture).

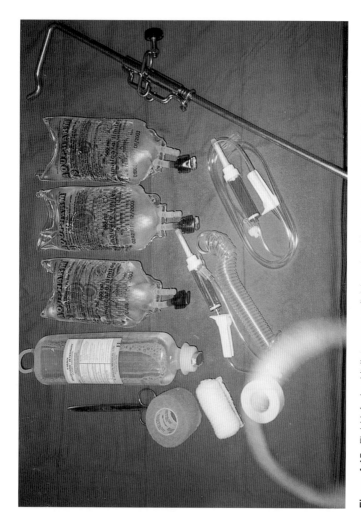

Figure 4.15. Fluid infusion kit (intravenous fluid packs, drip stand, infusion sets, bandages, tapes, scissors).

Fluid infusion kit

- fluid bag – for individual patient requirements
- infusion set or burette infusion set
- zinc oxide tapes
- drip stand
- infusion pump (optional)
- fluid infusion record card.

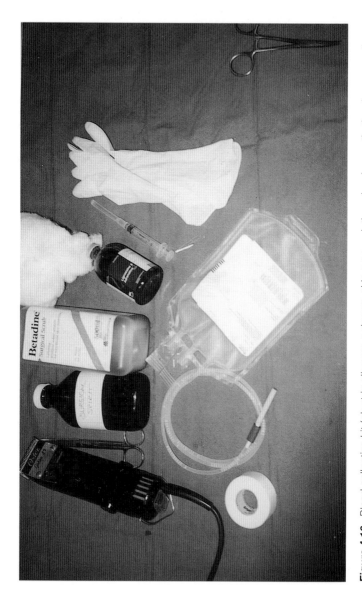

Figure 4.16. Blood collection kit (electric clippers, scissors, skin prep. solutions, local anaesthetic, gloves, needle and syringe, blood collection bag, tape and clamp).

Blood collection kit

- disposable apron and gloves
- local anaesthetic
- sterile 2 and 5 ml syringes
- sterile 23 g × 5/8 needle
- electric clippers
- surgical skin preparation solution (chlorhexidine or povidine iodine)
- surgical spirit
- scalpel blade size 10 or 11 (optional)
- blood collection bag – sodium citrate/acid citrate dextrose with correct amount of anticoagulant for volume of blood to be collected
- clamp to seal blood collection tube following collection
- needle holders, treves rat tooth forceps, suture needle and suture material to close venepuncture site (optional).

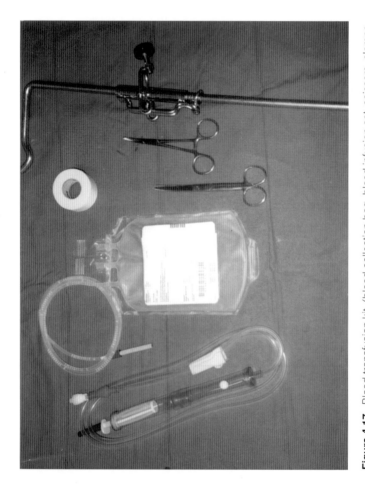

Figure 4.17. Blood transfusion kit (blood collection bag, blood infusion set, scissors, clamps, tape, drip stand).

Blood transfusion administration kit

- disposable apron and gloves
- electric clippers
- surgical skin preparation solution (chlorhexidine or povidine iodine)
- surgical spirit
- cotton wool swab
- scalpel blade (optional)
- zinc oxide tapes
- bung or three-way tap
- conforming bandage
- blood infusion set
- drip stand
- whole blood in sodium citrate collection bag (at body temperature)
- record card.

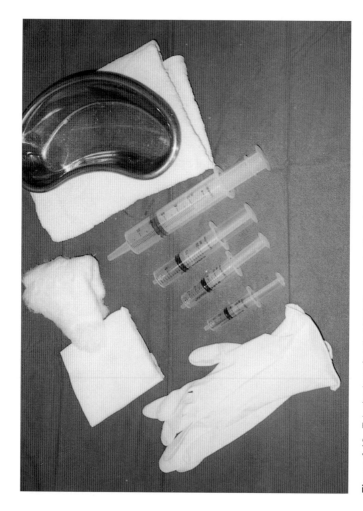

Figure 4.18. Tube/syringe feeding kit (gloves, selection of syringes, catheter and tip, cotton wool, swabs, towel, kidney bowl).

Assisted feeding kits

Syringe feeding kit

- disposable apron and gloves
- catheter tip syringe
- selection of syringes
- prewarmed food or fluid
- towel.

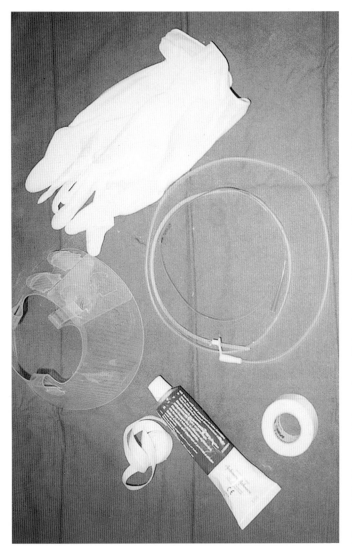

Figure 4.19. Naso-gastric/oesophageal tube placement (naso-gastric/oesophageal tubes, lubricant, gloves, Elizabethan collar, tape).

Tube feeding kit

- disposable apron and gloves
- assistant to restrain patient
- selected liquid diet or liquidized food
- selection of sterile syringes
- warm water to flush tube
- carbonated water (optional)
- calculated measured volume of food prewarmed (calculation see page 56)
- emollient cream to protect tube site
- paper and hand towel.

Naso-oesophageal tube placement kit

- disposable apron and gloves
- naso-oesophageal tube
- lubricating fluid/gel
- local anaesthetic spray
- tissue glue or suture kit to secure tube in place
- Elizabethan collar.

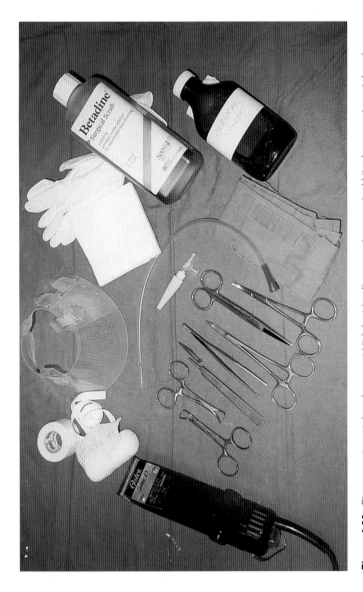

Figure 4.20.   Pharyngostomy tube placement kit (electric clippers, minor surgical kit, pharyngostomy tube, drape, skin prep. solutions, swabs, gloves, Elizabethan collar, tapes).

Pharyngostomy tube placement kit

- disposable apron and gloves
- electric clippers
- surgical skin preparation solution (chlorhexidine or povidine iodine)
- surgical spirit
- minor surgical kit (needle holders and stitch scissors, rat tooth forceps, spencer wells forceps, scalpel blade and handle, towel clips, suture needles and material)
- surgical drape
- pharyngostomy tube
- bung for pharyngostomy tube
- bandage
- Elizabethan collar.

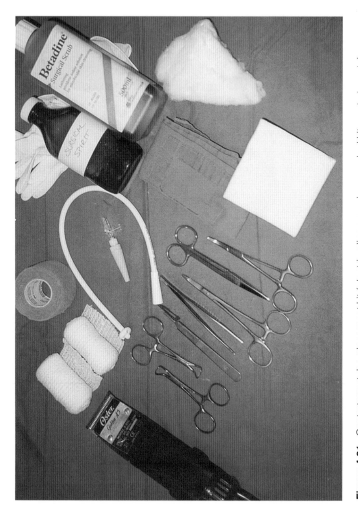

Figure 4.21. Gastrotomy tube placement kit (electric clippers, minor surgical kit, gastrotomy tube, drape, swabs, surgical skin prep. solutions, bandages, gloves).

Gastrotomy tube placement kit

Percutaneous endoscopic placement
- anaesthetized patient
- endoscope
- electric clippers
- surgical skin preparation solution (chlorhexidine or povidine iodine)
- surgical spirit
- minor surgical kit (needle holders and stitch scissors, Mayo scissors, rat tooth forceps, artery forceps, towel clips, suture needle and material, scalpel handle and blade)
- surgical drape
- sterile scrub assistant
- mushroom tipped gastrotomy tube
- suture material to secure placement
- conforming bandage or gauze
- Elizabethan collar.

Calculation

Fluid deficit and maintenance requirements

- Details
  - patient – 20 kg dog
  - clinical history – off food and water for 3 days and vomiting four times a day for the last 2 days
- Action
  - calculate insensible losses × 3 days (25 ml/kg/24 h × 20 kg) = 1500 ml
  - calculate sensible losses × 3 days (25 ml/kg/24 h × 20 kg × 1) = 500 ml (urine losses will be reduced due to lack of fluid intake)
  - calculate loss from vomiting four times a day (4 ml/kg/vomit × 20 × 2) = 640 ml
  - total fluid deficit = 1500 + 500 + 640 = 2640 ml.

Calculation of drip rate

- Daily maintenance infusion for 20 kg dog to be administered over an 8 h period
  - calculate daily maintenance fluid requirement for 20 kg dog at 50 ml/kg/24 h = 1250 ml/24 h
  - calculate volume of fluid to be given over 8 h – divide 1250 ml by 8 h = 156 ml/h
  - calculate volume of fluid to be given per minute – divide 156 ml by 60 min = 2.60 ml/min
  - infusion set delivers 20 drops/ml. Calculate the drips per minute – 2.60 ml × 20 = 52 drops
  - calculate drops per second – divide 52 drops by 60 = 0.8 drops/s (round up to one drop per second).

Calculation of energy requirements

1. Calculate daily resting energy requirement (RER) for over 5 kg bodyweight (bwt)
   Formula:

   $$RER = (30 \times kg\,bwt) + 70\,kcal$$

   e.g. to find RER for a 10 kg dog

   $$RER = (30 \times 10) + 70$$
   $$= 300 + 70$$
   $$= 370\,kcal/day$$

2. Calculate daily resting energy requirement (RER) for 5 kg bwt and under
   Formula:

   $$RER = (60 \times kg\,bwt) + 70\,kcal$$

   e.g. to find RER for a 3 kg cat

   $$RER = (60 \times 3) + 70$$
   $$= 180 + 70$$
   $$= 250\,kcal/day$$

3. Calculate illness energy requirement (IER) in relation to daily RER
   a. hospitalized/cage rest $= 1.2 \times RER$
   b. surgery/trauma $= 1.3 - 1.5 \times RER$
   c. cancer/sepsis $= 1.7 \times RER$
   d. burns $= 2 \times RER$

Calculation of food quantities to be administered

1. Calculate quantity of kcals to be fed to a hospitalized 10 kg dog

    a. 10 kg dog requires 370 kcal/day at rest
    = 370 (RER) × 1.2 (IER) for hospitalized patient
    = 444 kcal/day

2. Calculate quantity of food in millilitres to be fed to a 10 kg dog. Food value 1.5 kcal/ml

    a. Dog requires 444 kcal/day
    = 444 kcal divided by 1.5 kcal
    = 296 ml/day

3. Divide daily requirement into equal feeds to be administered throughout day

    a. 296 ml divided by eight feeds = 37 ml/feed

Drug percentage solutions

How to calculate a dose rate in millilitres of 2.5% thiopentone for a 20 kg dog at a dose rate of 25 mg/kg.

- 2.5% solution = 2.5 g/100 ml or 25 mg/ml
- 20 kg dog × dose rate of 25 mg/kg (20 × 25) = 500 mg
- drug strength is 25 mg/ml, therefore 500 mg divided by 25 mg = 20 ml
- dog requires 20 ml of 2.5% solution.

Drug dosage calculation

How to calculate the daily dose of an antibiotic for a 20 kg dog. The antibiotic is presented as 100 mg/ml. Drug dose rate for dogs is 22 mg/kg daily.

- 20 kg dog requires 22 mg/kg (20 × 22) = 440 mg
- antibiotic presented as 100 mg/1 ml; 10 mg/0.1 ml
- 440 mg divided by 100 mg = 4.4 ml
- dog requires 4.4 ml of antibiotic solution daily.

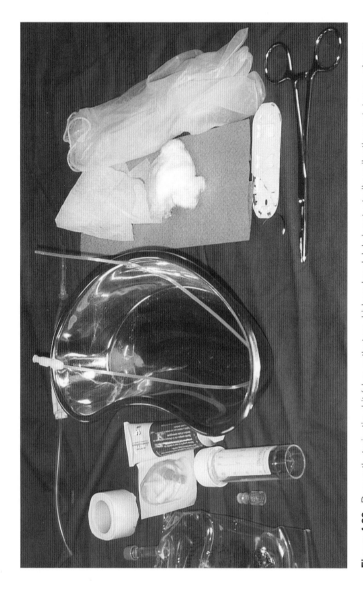

Figure 4.22. Dog catheterization kit (dog catheters, kidney bowl, lubricant, sterile collection pot, tapes, gloves, urine collection bag, suture equipment).

Urinary catheterization kits

Dog catheterization kit

- disposable apron and gloves
- assistant to help restrain as required
- sterile kidney dish
- sterile urinary collection pot
- lubricant
- disposable absorbable paper
- swabs
- sterile dog catheter of appropriate size
- syringe, three-way tap, bung/urine collection bag as required
- suture material, zinc oxide tape and Elizabethan collar (if indwelling)
- suture kit.

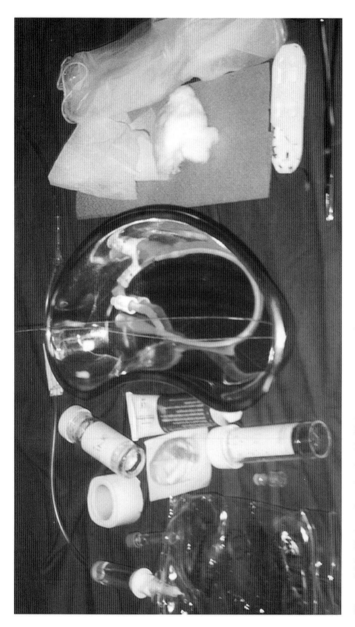

Figure 4.23. Bitch catheterization kit (Foley catheter, water for injection, urine collection pot and bag, lubricant, gloves, kidney bowl, suture equipment).

Bitch catheterization kit

- disposable apron and gloves
- assistant to help restrain as required
- sterile kidney dish
- sterile urinary collection pot
- lubricant
- speculum and light source as required
- disposable absorbable paper
- swabs
- sterile catheter of appropriate size and type, e.g. Foley, Tiemanns
- syringe, three-way tap, bung/urine collection bag as required
- suture material (dependent on catheter type), zinc oxide tape and Elizabethan collar (if indwelling).

If a Foley catheter is being used the following will also be required:

- stylet
- saline/sterile water for cuff inflation.

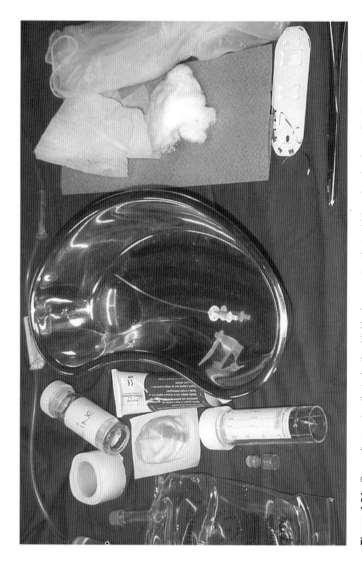

Figure 4.24. Queen/tom cat catheterization kit (Jackson cat catheter, kidney bowl, urine collection pot and bag, lubricant, gloves, suture equipment, three-way tap).

Tom cat catheterization kit

- disposable apron and gloves
- assistant to help restrain as required
- sterile kidney dish
- sterile urinary collection pot
- lubricant
- disposable absorbable paper
- sterile cat catheter of appropriate size, e.g. Jackson
- syringe, three-way tap, bung/urine collection bag as required
- suture material, zinc oxide tape and Elizabethan collar (if indwelling).

Queen catheterization kit

- disposable apron and gloves
- assistant to help restrain as required
- sterile kidney dish
- sterile urinary collection pot
- lubricant
- disposable absorbable paper
- sterile cat catheter of appropriate size
- syringe, three-way tap, bung/urine collection bag as required.

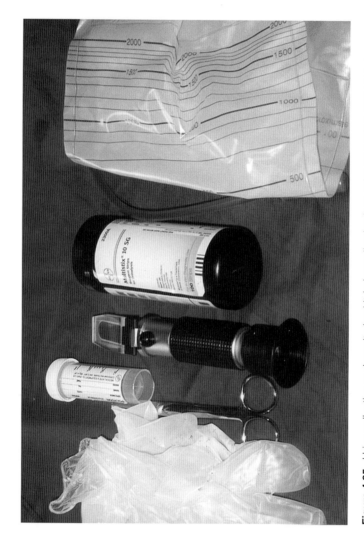

Figure 4.25. Urine collection and monitoring kit (urine collection bag, urine test strips, refractometer, sterile collection pot, gloves, scissors).

Urine collection and monitoring kit

After indwelling catheterization
- disposable apron and gloves
- urine collection bag
- spigot/bung (as appropriate to catheter)
- sterile urine collection pot
- refractometer (if measurement required)
- urinary dipsticks (if measurement required)
- record card.

NB. *Measurement of urine volume is likely to be required. Ensure that measurement can be read from the urinary collection bag or include a syringe to measure manually.*

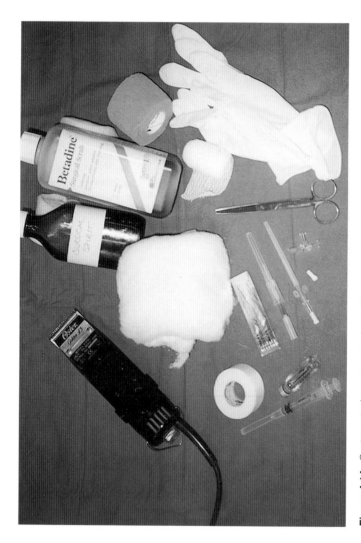

Figure 4.14. Cystocentesis, paracentesis and thoracentesis kit (skin prep. solutions, gloves, scissors, electric clippers, intravenous catheters, heparinized saline, cotton wool). Also suitable for IV access.

Aspiration of fluids

Cystocentesis, paracentesis, thoracocentesis kits (see Figure 4.14)

- disposable apron and gloves
- assistant to help restrain as required
- electric clippers
- skin preparation equipment
- appropriate needle and syringe
- three-way tap
- sterile kidney dish
- sample collection pots as required
- local anaesthetic.

NB. *A thoracic drain may be used for longer-term thoracocentesis.*

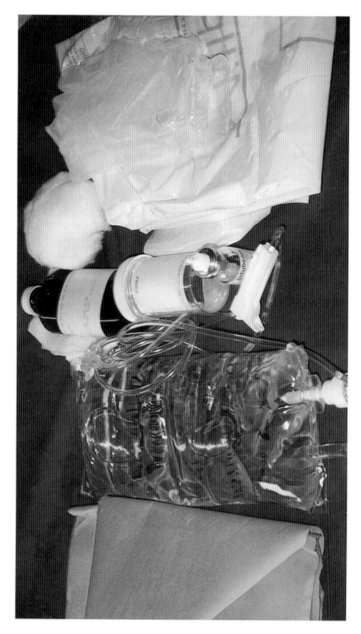

Figure 4.26. Peritoneal dialysis kit (drape, dialysis fluid, local anaesthetic, skin prep. solutions, gloves, apron).

Peritoneal dialysis kit

- disposable apron and gloves
- assistant to help restrain as required
- electric clippers
- skin preparation equipment
- local anaesthetic
- small surgical pack and drapes
- peritoneal catheter
- giving set
- dialysis fluid (warmed to body temperature)
- sample collection pot as required.

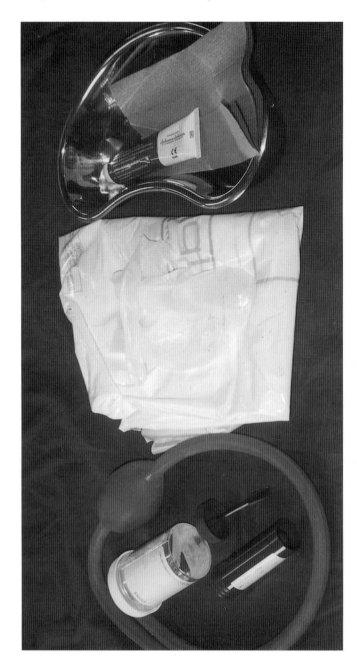

Figure 4.27. Enema administration kit (Higginsons syringe, faeces collection pot, gloves, apron, lubricant, kidney bowl).

Enema administration kit

It is advisable to administer an enema to a dog whilst adjacent to an outside exit to allow for immediate defecation.

- disposable apron and gloves
- absorbable paper
- lubricant
- fluid receptacle of appropriate size
- proprietary enema/enema solution
- Higginsons syringe/can and tubing as required
- faecal collection pot if required
- clinical waste bin adjacent.

NB. *A clean litter tray should be available in the kennel of a cat that has had an enema.*

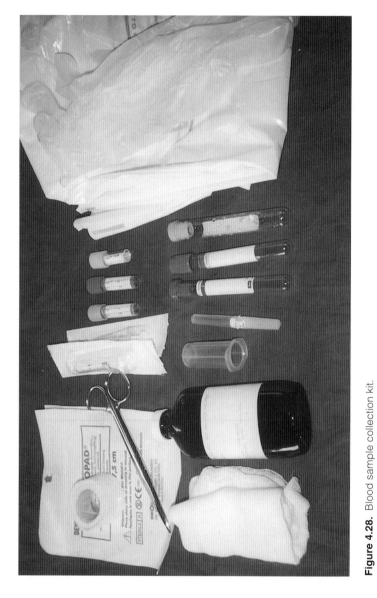

Figure 4.28. Blood sample collection kit.

Collection of samples

Blood sample collection kit

- disposable apron and gloves
- swab
- antiseptic solution
- assistant to raise vein and restrain animal
- basic dressing

either:

- needle (of appropriate size, i.e. as large a gauge as possible)
- syringe (of appropriate size, i.e. for the amount to be collected)
- appropriate sample tube

or:

- vacutainer double ended needle
- vacutainer holder
- vacutainer tube (appropriate for sample to be taken).

Table 4.1. Choice of blood tubes

Colour	Anticoagulant	Sample type
White	None	Serum
Pink	EDTA	Whole blood/plasma
Yellow	Oxalate fluoride	Whole blood/plasma
Orange	Heparin	Whole blood/plasma
Purple	Sodium citrate	Whole blood/plasma

Table 4.2. Choice of vacutainer tubes

Colour	Anticoagulant	Sample type
Red	None	Serum
Lavender	EDTA	Whole blood/plasma
Grey	Oxalate fluoride	Whole blood/plasma
Orange/green	Heparin	Whole blood/plasma
Purple	Sodium citrate	Whole blood/plasma

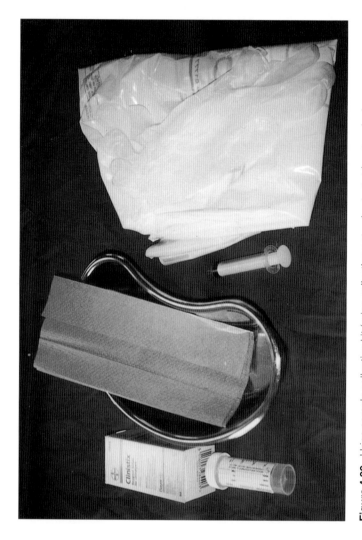

Figure 4.29. Urine sample collection kit (urine collection pot, urine test strips, towel, gloves, apron, syringe, kidney bowl).

Urine sample collection kit

- disposable apron and gloves
- sterilized kidney dish
- syringe
- universal container
- assistant to restrain animal if required
- refrigeration facilities.

NB. *Urine may be collected after voluntary voiding, via gentle pressure on the bladder or by urethral catheterization (see pages 59–65). Preservatives may be required for some external testing. Contact your external laboratory for details as to requirements.*

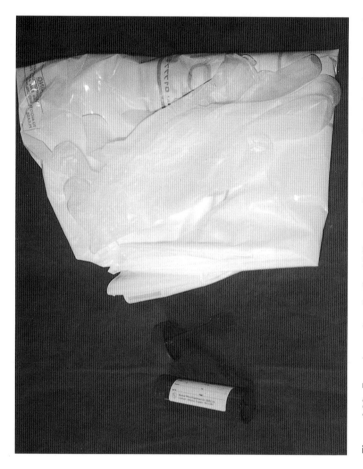

Figure 4.30. Faecal sample collection kit (faeces collection pot and spatula, gloves, apron).

Faecal sample collection kit

- disposable apron and gloves
- assistant to restrain patient as required
- faecal pot or wide-mouthed universal container
- transport swab – if testing is to be delayed
- refrigeration facilities.

NB. *If possible, collect faeces directly from the rectum using a gloved finger and fill the pot.*

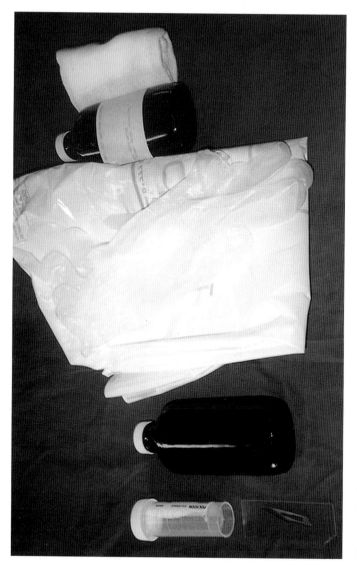

Figure 4.31. Skin scrape collection kit (collection pot, scalpel blade, paraffin oil, gloves, apron, microscope slide).

Skin scrape kit

- disposable gloves and apron
- paraffin oil
- microscope slides
- scalpel blade
- universal container
- refrigeration facilities
- saline/antiseptic preparation
- swabs.

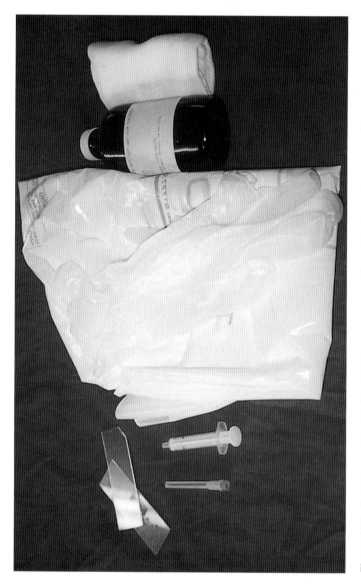

Figure 4.32.   Pustule sample collection kit (gloves, apron, needle and syringe, microscope slides, spreader slide).

Pustule sample kit

- disposable apron and gloves
- sterile needle
- 1–2 ml syringe
- microscope slide
- spreader slide
- universal container
- transport swab.

NB. *Examine sample whilst fresh.*

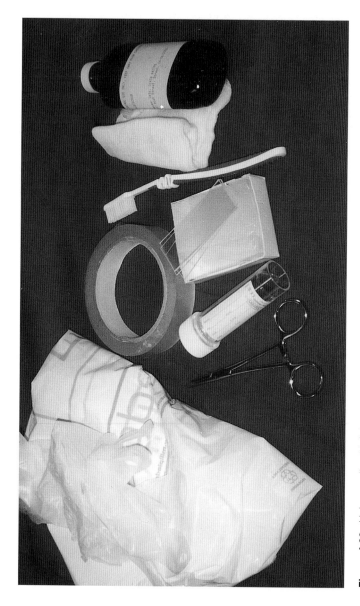

Figure 4.33. Hair sampling kit (gloves, apron, brush, forceps, clear adhesive tape, universal container, microscope slides).

Hair sampling kit

To enable collection by plucking, taping or brushing.

- disposable apron and gloves
- clear adhesive tape
- forceps
- small bristle brush (toothbrush)
- microscope slides
- universal container/Petri dish
- saline/antiseptic preparation
- swabs.

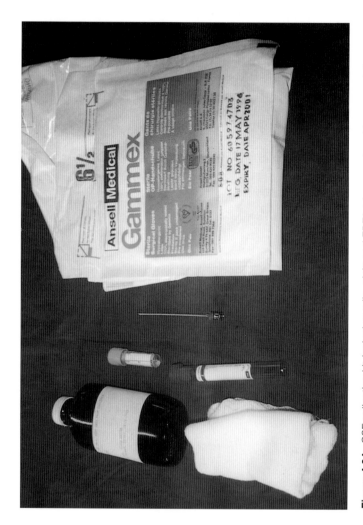

Figure 4.34. CSF collection kit (spinal needle, plain and EDTA tubes, swabs, skin prep. solution, drapes, gloves, apron).

Cerebrospinal fluid collection kit

- disposable apron and gloves
- electric clippers
- antiseptic skin preparation
- swabs
- sterile gloves
- sterile spinal tap needle
- EDTA tube
- plain tube.

NB. *Fluid to be collected by thoraco or paracentesis or from synovial joints will require the same equipment with the addition of appropriate hypodermic needles replacing the spinal tap needle.*

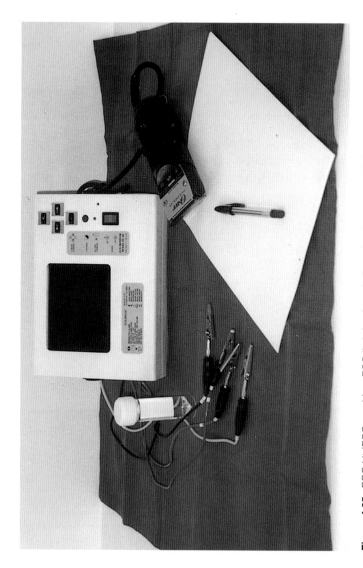

Figure 4.35. ECG kit (ECG machine, ECG limb leads and clips, electric clippers, ECG gel, paper and pen for recordings).

Diagnostic procedure kits

Electrocardiography kit

- assistant to restrain patient
- quiet environment
- electric clippers
- ECG machine
- leads and clips
- electrical supply
- electrode gel
- recording paper
- pen for labelling recording.

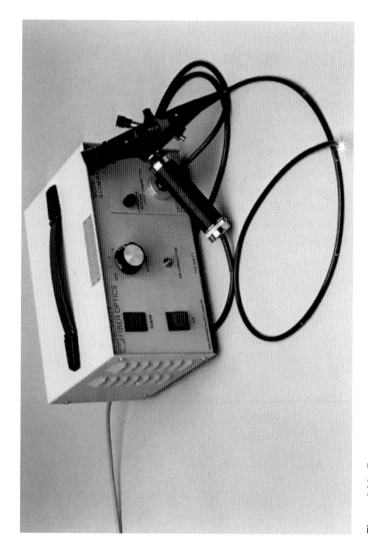

Figure 4.36. Endoscopy kit.

Endoscopy kit

- assistant
- endoscope
- light source
- biopsy attachments (as required)
- lubricant
- normal saline
- catheter.

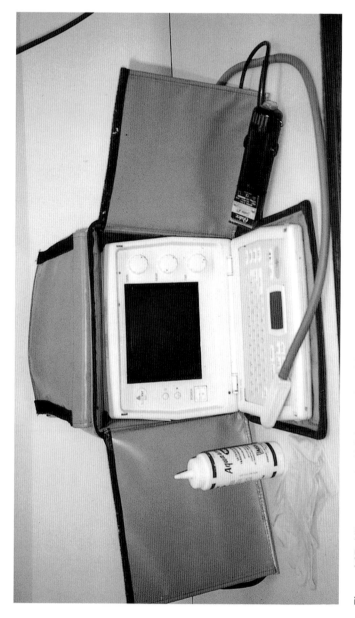

Figure 4.37. Ultrasonography kit (ultrasound machine, transducer gel, electric clippers).

Ultrasonography kit

- assistant to restrain patient
- electric clippers
- ultrasound machine
- monitor
- transducers
- electrical supply
- coupling gel
- printer
- paper.

5
Self-assessment

Crossword

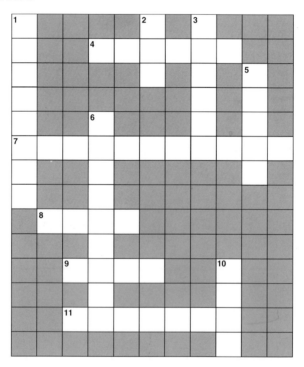

Across

4. Transports disease
7. Measures heat
8. Keep firm
9. Tracheostomy .....
11. Prevents clotting

Down

1. Use to collect urine
2. Investigates heart
3. Inanimate object
5. Bitch catheter
6. Give blood
10. Plug

How well do you score on medical kits?

Multiple choice

1. The ideal **intravenous catheter** size for the cephalic vein of a feline neonate would be:
   (a) 18 g
   (b) 20 g
   (c) 22 g
   (d) 24 g

2. The daily maintenance **fluid requirement** for a healthy dog is:
   (a) 10–20 ml/kg/24 h
   (b) 25–35 ml/kg/24 h
   (c) 40–50 ml/kg/24 h
   (d) 55–65 ml/kg/24 h

3. The **anticoagulant** used for blood collected for transfusion is:
   (a) lithium heparin
   (b) fluoride oxalate
   (c) sodium citrate
   (d) EDTA

4. The **ideal catheter** suitable for gastrotomy tube placement is:
   (a) Foley
   (b) Tiemanns
   (c) Jackson
   (d) mushroom

5. The **minimum** acceptable urine output of a healthy adult dog per kg bodyweight per hour is:
   (a) 1–2 ml
   (b) 3–4 ml
   (c) 5–6 ml
   (d) 7–8 ml

6. The **temperature** of a healthy adult cat should be:
   (a) 30–37°C
   (b) 38–38.5°C
   (c) 30–37°F
   (d) 38–38.5°F

7. The resting energy requirement **(RER)** for a healthy 20 kg dog is:
   (a) 200–300 kcal/day
   (b) 400–500 kcal/day
   (c) 600–700 kcal/day
   (e) 800–900 kcal/day

8. The illness energy requirement **(IER)** for a 10 kg dog with burns is:
   (a) 440 kcal/day
   (b) 540 kcal/day
   (c) 640 kcal/day
   (d) 740 kcal/day

9. The resting energy requirement **(RER)** for a healthy 4.5 kg cat is:
   (a) 100–200 kcal/day
   (b) 210–300 kcal/day
   (c) 310–400 kcal/day
   (d) 410–500 kcal/day

10. The strength in mg/ml of a drug with a **percentage solution** of 7.5% is:
    (a) 0.75
    (b) 7.5
    (c) 75
    (d) 750

11. An example of a **zoonotic disease** is:
    (a) adenovirus
    (b) bordetella bronchiseptica
    (c) leptospirosis
    (d) parvovirus

12. The type of 'gel' useful for **ultrasonography** is:
    (a) coupling
    (b) electrode
    (c) obstetrical
    (d) lubricant

13. The type of **catheter** routinely used to catheterize tom cats is the:
    (a) Tiemanns
    (b) Jackson
    (c) Foley
    (d) metal

14. A vacutainer tube containing **EDTA** as an anticoagulant is coloured:
    (a) red
    (b) grey
    (c) orange
    (d) lavender

15. The type of acid **NOT** used as preservative for urine is:
    (a) citric
    (b) boric
    (c) hydrochloric
    (d) acetic

Answer Key

¹C					²E		³F			
A			⁴V	E	C	T	O	R		
T					G		M		⁵F	
H							I		O	
E			⁶T				T		L	
⁷T	H	E	R	M	O	M	E	T	E	R
E			A						Y	
R			N							
	⁸C	A	S	T						
			F							
		⁹T	U	B	E			¹⁰B		
			S					U		
		¹¹H	E	P	A	R	I	N		
								G		

Across

4. Transports disease
7. Measures heat
8. Keep firm
9. Tracheostomy .....
11. Prevents clotting

Down

1. Use to collect urine
2. Investigates heart
3. Inanimate object
5. Bitch catheter
6. Give blood
10. Plug

Answers

1. d	6. b	11. c
2. c	7. c	12. a
3. c	8. d	13. b
4. d	9. c	14. d
5. a	10. c	15. a

6
Selected reading

Aspinall, V. (In press) *Clinical Procedures in Veterinary Nursing.* Elsevier Science, Oxford (ISBN 0750654163).

Bowden, C. and Masters, J. (In press) *Textbook of Medical Veterinary Nursing.* Elsevier Science, Oxford (ISBN 0750651717).

Lane, D. R. and Cooper, B. (1999) *Veterinary Nursing*, 2nd ed. Butterworth-Heinemann, Oxford (ISBN 0750639997).

Orpet, H. and Welsh, P. (2001) *Handbook of Veterinary Nursing.* Blackwell Science, Oxford (ISBN 0632052589).

Index